> *In our country, the lie has become not just a moral category but a pillar of the state. In breaking with the lie we are performing a moral act, not a political one, not one that can be punished by criminal law, but one that would immediately have an effect on our way of life.*

> ALEKSANDR SOLZHENITSYN
> *Russian writer and Nobel Peace Prize winner,*
> *January 1974*

On December 1, 2019, a man in Wuhan, China, suffering from flu-like symptoms for several days was admitted to a hospital for what would be diagnosed as a severe form of pneumonia. His fate is unknown.

For thirty days the Chinese Communist Party (CCP) took no action to alert the world of the impending danger of a deadly new disease. Those thirty days shook the world.

A Marxist-Leninist regime that was built on the bodies of 60 million Chinese since its founding in 1949 lied to the world and

Why have American scientists not demanded a full accounting from Beijing for its bat coronavirus research?

repressed medical doctors who tried to warn of a new highly contagious virus.

In the days ahead, tens of thousands of people would die, and the entire world would be thrown into economic chaos.

This is nothing less than a crime against humanity facilitated by CCP influence within the World Health Organization (WHO), a United Nations agency with the primary mission of preparing to fight just the kind of disease outbreak that took place. The WHO and its leadership turned out to be worse than useless during the single crisis for which the agency exists. Instead, the WHO served as an agent for spreading dangerously false information by the CCP.

U.S. President Donald Trump vowed to cut off the United States's annual $400 million in funding for the WHO as the epidemic forced the shutdown of the American and global economies in a bid to mitigate the spread of the disease.

"The world is shut down," the president said. "Nobody has ever seen anything like this. The entire world is shut down."

Only Information Age communications that emerged within the nearly totalitarian control system in China prevented the CCP from completely covering up the epidemic and perhaps inflicting even greater global damage.

Social media posts by Wuhan doctors sounded the alarm early on in the crisis. The clues allowed Western intelligence agencies to pick up the first signs. A brief period of time during the earliest days also allowed official and unofficial media to reveal what was going on. That was abruptly shut down in January when the CCP imposed harsh censorship and restrictions, including jailing unofficial bloggers in Wuhan who were telling the world of the horrors inflicted upon a city of 11 million people.

The party under Xi Jinping and his functionaries, from the highest levels in Beijing down to local officials in Wuhan, lied and deceived their own people. Then they launched a campaign of deception and disinformation. They failed to inform the world of the outbreak of a deadly new disease caused by a new coronavirus derived from bats, animals that were the subject of extensive research after the first outbreak in 2003 of the disease called Severe Acute Respiratory Syndrome (SARS). The new virus is called SARS-Coronavirus-2 (SARS-CoV-2).

After first covering up the outbreak by attributing it to poor sanitary conditions at a wild animal market in Wuhan, Chinese authorities launched a disinformation campaign asserting that the virus had originated outside China. Official propaganda mouthpieces said the virus was created in the United States and spread by U.S. Army soldiers who attended a military sporting competition in Wuhan in October 2019.

President Trump and Secretary of State Mike Pompeo denied the lies but did not condemn them over fears that China was preparing to pull out of a landmark trade agreement with the United States that requires China to purchase $250 billion in American goods. The president and senior officials exposed the campaign as a desperate effort by Beijing to deflect international attention from its criminal mishandling of the virus outbreak.

The People's Republic of China and the CCP that has ruled it with an iron fist since 1949 carried out the cover-up in a premeditated fashion. Like the Soviet Union that spawned it, the CCP was built, as the Russian writer Aleksander Solzhenitsyn said of the Soviet Union, on lies and deception. It thrived on lies and has held on to power with lies.

Communist leaders constantly harp on bogus assertions that China is mistreated by the international community and is not recognized as a great nation. The truth is that the damage the CCP has inflicted upon the world proves without a doubt that the institution is a force for evil that must be replaced with a new and open system of government.

For the United States, the CCP has shown through its missteps that anything related to it – its representatives, its controlled businesses, its fellow travelers, and its apologists – should no longer be welcome inside free Western institutions built on trust.

As part of a strategy of seeking global supremacy under Xi's Chinese Dream, the CCP is exploiting the global health crisis to advance its agenda. For Beijing, achieving global supremacy is intimately linked to seeking the ultimate destruction of the United States of America – the main obstacle to that goal.

THE OUTBREAK

The Wuhan Municipal Center for Disease Control and Prevention is located about three miles from what many Chinese and American scientists believe is the epicenter of the virus outbreak – one of the many notorious wild animal markets. The Wuhan Huanan Seafood Wholesale Market is a source of exotic fresh meat from animals such as civet cats and pangolins, scaly anteaters considered delicacies by China's ruling elites.

The Wuhan CDC is home to a laboratory staffed by a researcher named Tian Junhua. Tian burst into prominence in China in December 2019 just as the deadly coronavirus was attacking its first victims. State-controlled propaganda outlets, both print and video, lionized Tian as a dedicated researcher committed to finding vaccines for deadly bat coronaviruses. He was shown wearing protective gear inside caves in China, catching bats and taking swabs from their mouths.

The documentary revealed that Tian at one point in his field research was exposed to bat urine inside a cave because he had failed to wear protective gear. To avoid contracting a disease, the researcher self-quarantined for fourteen days – the same time period now being used around the world to protect people exposed to the new coronavirus. How did Tian know that the possible incubation period for a SARS-like bat virus to infect a person was fourteen days? What kind of research was he doing on deadly bat coronaviruses at the CDC's Level 2 security laboratory, a facility lacking the kind of equipment needed for handling deadly pathogens? Was he working on the recently discovered bat coronavirus now dubbed SARS-COV-2?

These and other questions remain unanswered by the CCP. And many in the international scientific community appear to be running interference for the party by dismissing all public discussion about Chinese laboratory research on bat coronaviruses as a conspiracy theory.

Army General Mark Milley, chairman of the Joint Chiefs of Staff, insists that the idea of the virus leaking from an unsecure Chinese laboratory is no conspiracy theory. "It should be no surprise that we've taken a keen interest in that, and we've had a lot of intelligence [agencies] take a hard look at that," he said. "I would just say at this point it's inconclusive, although the weight of evidence seems to indicate natural. But we don't know for certain."

The remarks to reporters in April were the first time a senior American leader had disclosed that the deadly virus may have escaped from a Chinese laboratory.

The market China claimed was the source of the outbreak remained open throughout December despite doctors in Wuhan linking the outbreak there.

State Department cables from January 2018 revealed that American scientific diplomats issued several warnings about the lack of security at the Wuhan Institute of Virology.

One of the cables, publicized by the *Washington Post*, disclosed a "serious shortage" of trained personnel at the institute's new French-built lab that were needed to "safely operate this high-containment laboratory."

The origin of the virus remains couched in CCP secrecy. Chinese government spokesmen sidestep questions about the virus's origin by saying the question is a matter for scientists to investigate. Why then has no action been taken by Chinese authorities? And why have American scientists not demanded a full accounting from Beijing for its bat coronavirus research? The silence has raised suspicions that the CCP has played a malevolent role in the crisis.

For several weeks in early 2020, the disease was called Wuhan pneumonia throughout China. Then in March 2020, Chinese Communist Party authorities realized the use of the city name was fueling the growing international outrage and resentment toward the People's Republic of China that for a second time since 2003 was inflicting a deadly global disease outbreak on the world.

Using its political influence, the CCP pressured the WHO to give the disease the more technically neutral name COVID-19, short for "coronavirus disease 2019."

In 2003, SARS created the first Chinese pandemic as a result of a bat coronavirus. Although the origins of that virus also remain murky, the official explanation for that outbreak was that somehow the microbe had made the leap from cave-hanging nocturnal mammals into humans, possibly through a civet, one of the wild animal meat market delicacies.

The pandemic in 2003 was less devastating than the coronavirus crisis now spreading around the globe. It turns out that the new virus has a unique feature: those infected can easily spread it for a period up to fourteen days without symptoms.

The new coronavirus outbreak that began in Wuhan mushroomed into a deadly epidemic throughout China and then spread to the rest of the world. It struck with a vengeance not seen since the influenza pandemic in 1918 that claimed the lives of at least 50 million people.

By April 10, 2020, more than 1.6 million people had tested positive, with a death count of nearly 100,000 people.

U.S. intelligence agencies believe the Chinese lied about the numbers of people infected and those who had died, that the true numbers are orders of magnitude larger. An analysis by Derek Scissors, a scholar at the American Enterprise Institute, estimates that at least 2.9 million people were stricken in China alone, causing at least 136,000 deaths.

It is important that blame for the current crisis be placed squarely at the feet of the ruling CCP, an institution that has perpetuated its reviled rule for decades through a combination of raw power and repression. It is backed by the connivance of foreign politicians, business leaders, and journalists who refuse to recognize the inherent evil of the Chinese communist system. The fawning over this revolutionary anti-American regime is similar to liberal progressive praise for the Soviet Union until its collapse in 1991.

If there could be a single bright spot amid the death and disruption caused by the coronavirus pandemic, it is that this incident has laid bare the dangers of continued economic and political engagement with the CCP.

It is now clear the United States must shake off any past delusions about the so-called Chinese economic miracle – a success story built largely on the massive theft of American technology. America must clearly recognize that Communist China today poses the most significant threat to world peace, freedom, and stability. Further, now is the time to declare that the only solution to the problem is for the Chinese Communist Party, like its progenitor the Soviet Union, to be quickly dispatched to the dustbin of history, as the great American President Ronald Reagan once said of that earlier evil empire.

December 1, 2020, marked the day the

first known case of COVID-19 was discovered. It was revealed by a group of twenty-nine Chinese scientists writing in the British medical journal *The Lancet*. Another news outlet, the Chinese government-controlled *Caixin*, dates the first case to December 15. The *Wall Street Journal*, before its cadre of reporters was ousted from China, provided further details and linked the first known case to December 10.

Around the same time as that first reported case, another man presented at a Wuhan hospital with pneumonia-like symptoms. The man would be the first of several cases linked by authorities to the Huanan Seafood Wholesale Market. Five days later, his wife caught the disease. The couple provided the first clue that the highly contagious virus could be transmitted between people.

This is one of the most important reasons the pandemic is directly caused by the Chinese Communist Party. It was the most important piece of information that could have prevented global devastation.

In *The Lancet*, the twenty-nine Chinese scientists examined what were suggested as the first forty-one victims of the coronavirus, including the first patient who became ill on December 1. The paper notes that the research was funded by the Chinese Ministry of Science and Technology, the Chinese Academy of Medical Sciences, the National Natural Science Foundation of China, and the Beijing Municipal Science and Technology Commission. The authors were doctors from Jinyintan Hospital in Wuhan that handled the forty-one cases.

The study became a key part of the CCP's

Trusting false Chinese data in the early days of this crisis has been lethal for countries foolish enough to do so, including the United States.

initial propaganda campaign about the virus outbreak – that the disease began at the market. Yet the study also contained the seeds that would eventually unravel the market origin theory of the virus.

According to the study, most of the first patients stricken with the disease had a "shared history of exposure to Huanan seafood market" – the wet market that trafficked in exotic animals. Thus, the scientists were pointing to the food market as the problem and away from the nearby Wuhan Municipal CDC, where bat coronaviruses were being worked on in a laboratory ill-prepared to prevent an inadvertent leak or infection.

Gao Fu, director of the Chinese Center for Disease Control and Prevention, told state-controlled media that initial signs indicated the virus had originated from wild animals sold at a seafood market. Yet the January study proved one thing: the virus source was not limited to the wild animal market. In fact, of the first four known patients studied who became ill between December 1 and December 10, three of them had no contact with the market, including the first patient. In fact, the first patient linked to the market was not detected until December 10, further raising doubts about the theory.

From December 10 to December 14, no patients were infected. On December 15, two people became sick. Over the following five days, a total of ten people – all linked to the market – became ill. In all, fourteen of the forty-one patients studied had no connection to the market. It is possible they were infected by people who had been to the market. But without more information from the Chinese scientists, skepticism is called for.

"It is imperative that we identify the origin of the SARS CoV-2 virus," said Robert G. Darling, a medical doctor and expert on biological weapons formerly with the Army Medical Research Institute of Infectious Diseases at Fort Detrick, Maryland, and now chief medical officer for Patronus Medical. "The Chinese almost certainly know, but they have not shared it. By learning its origin, it will better help us understand the biology of the virus and how it behaves."

The Lancet said the following about the first patient diagnosed on December 1: "None of his family members developed fever or any respiratory symptoms. No epidemiological link was found between the first patient and later cases. The first fatal case, who had continuous exposure to the market, was admitted to hospital because of a 7-day history of fever, cough, and dyspnea [breathing difficulty]. Five days after illness onset, his wife, a 53-year-old woman who had no known history of exposure to the market, also presented with pneumonia and was hospitalized in the isolation ward."

Curiously, the Chinese study did not list the date when the information was known, and *The Lancet* said the report was "corrected" but did not identify the correction.

The December 1 patient was an elderly man who suffered from dementia. "He lived four or five buses [stops] from the seafood market, and because he was sick he basically didn't go out," Wu Wenjuan, a senior doctor at Wuhan's Jinyintan Hospital and one of the authors of the study, told the BBC.

Wu told a slightly different story to the *Wall Street Journal*, telling the newspaper that the first case appeared on December 12 when a forty-nine-year-old vendor at the market fell ill and that seven days later his father-in-law became sick.

Did the CCP change its story because the first patient was not linked to the market?

The Wuhan government provided still another date. Communist authorities said the first patient infected showed symptoms on December 8, along with a relative who fell ill several days later.

A chart in the *Lancet* study, however, shows no cases of the disease surfacing between December 10 and December 15, further confusing exactly when the first cases surfaced.

The *South China Morning Post*, a Hong Kong newspaper owned by the Chinese government–controlled Alibaba technology company, reported seeing documents listing the first patient infection as November 17 — two weeks before the official first case. That report has not been confirmed, and claiming a November starting point could be deliberately false information designed to fit what I will show later was the CCP's disinformation campaign to blame the United States for causing the outbreak.

None of the early cases are believed to be the elusive Patient Zero, the first person infected by the disease that virus investigators must identify and locate if the precise origin of the coronavirus is to be determined. The CCP must be pressured by the international community to reveal what it knows.

THE VIRUS

As noted, the incubation period is between three and fourteen days. That is the time between when a person is infected and the first symptoms appear. Victims who become ill start out with aches and pains in the legs, arms, and back, together with a fever around

101 degrees. Other frequent early symptoms are a dry cough and difficulty breathing. If the first people infected showed up at Wuhan hospitals between December 1 and 15, that places the first infection – Patient Zero – at some time between November 15 and December 1.

On January 2, the Wuhan Institute of Virology completed its mapping of the genome for the deadly virus, but the breakthrough was not made public by the CCP.

The virus is believed to have been living quietly among China's horseshoe bat population for thousands of years until suddenly, mysteriously, it mutated.

No one at this point knows how the virus transferred from bats to a new host, whether human or animal. Like its brother, the SARS virus that is believed to have been transferred from bats to civets, the new virus may have been passed from a bat to a pangolin, a scaly anteater often sold in wet markets. However, Chinese authorities have produced no evidence that pangolins were sold at the Huanan Seafood Wholesale Market. Thus, a laboratory

There are no caves containing Horseshoe bats within five hundred miles of Wuhan.

leak through an infected worker or a corrupt lab employee who may have sold an infected animal to the market must be considered.

Jonathan Epstein, an epidemiologist at the EcoHealth Alliance in New York, has studied bat coronaviruses in China linked to SARS. He told the *New Yorker* that he was part of a team in China that discovered four species of bats that carried coronaviruses similar to SARS, including one that was more than a 90 percent match with the original SARS virus. Epstein said tests conducted by Chinese health authorities on animals at the Huanan market showed no signs of the new coronavirus. The exact animals tested at the market, however, were not specified. Later, authorities claimed to have found the new virus in samples obtained from the market's tables and gutters.

One of the most important figures in the mystery surrounding the deadly pandemic is a colleague of Epstein's, a medical researcher known as Shi Zheng-Li, who has come to be known in China as "the Bat Woman of Wuhan" for her research on bat viruses.

Shi, a scientist at the Key Laboratory of Special Pathogens and Biosafety at the Wuhan Institute of Virology, remains a key figure in the ongoing viral disease outbreak, and questions about her role in it have circulated among millions of people in China.

The social media scrutiny prompted her to go public with an unusual comment denying her laboratory had anything to do with the outbreak. She insists the virus was the result of a natural mutation and not a release from her laboratory. "The 2019 novel coronavirus is a punishment by nature to humans' unsanitary lifestyle," she said on her WeChat account on February 2. "I promise with my life that the virus has nothing to do with the lab."

In 2015, Shi joined nine other scientists in publishing a paper on laboratory work related to SARS and the danger that bat coronaviruses could infect humans. The paper published in *Nature* revealed that "we built a chimeric virus encoding a novel, zoonotic CoV spike protein ... isolated from Chinese horseshoe bats."

"The hybrid virus allowed us to evaluate the ability of the novel spike protein to cause disease independently of other necessary adaptive mutations in its natural backbone," Shi and the others added.

The statement is a clear indication that scientists had been engaged in laboratory manipulation of bat coronaviruses to determine how the microbes use special receptor cells that permit them to latch on to human cells and cause infections.

That research paper was published under the ominous headline, "A SARS-like cluster of circulating bat coronaviruses shows potential for human emergence."

The potential became a reality in December 2019 in Wuhan.

An even more alarming piece of evidence on the origin of the virus was produced by Shi and coauthor Zhou Peng in a paper submitted to the journal *Viruses* on January 29, 2020, and published two months later. The paper predicted that "it is highly likely that future SARS- or MERS-like coronavirus outbreaks will originate from bats, and there is an increased probability that this will occur in China." MERS is the Middle East Respiratory Syndrome that afflicted the Middle East beginning in 2012 and is caused by a bat coronavirus.

After Western news reports revealed China's extensive research on bat coronaviruses, the CCP cracked down. New restrictions were imposed in March 2020 on all scientific studies on the origin of the new coronavirus – a clear sign that Beijing is hiding details about the source of the pandemic.

By March 2020, global research underway

around the world on the new virus produced other startling results. In particular, a team of researchers writing in *Nature* stated that the new virus did not need to pass first to an animal host, unlike with the 2002–2004 SARS outbreak.

"Are intermediate hosts involved in the potential bat-to-human transmission of SARS-CoV-2?" the researchers asked. Their answer: because another bat coronavirus is closely related to the new virus that can directly infect humans, "one possibility is that there is not an intermediate host."

Epstein noted on Twitter that the study provided important insights about direct bat-to-human transmission. The authors also studied the possible jump from bats to pangolins to humans, but their main conclusion was that "an intermediate host for #SARS CoV2 is not necessary. This underscores importance of continued research to identify a #bat reservoir," Epstein tweeted.

According to authorities in China and people who worked there, no bats were sold at the Huanan Seafood Wholesale Market, thus further raising doubts about the official story that the virus started at the market.

Additionally, there are no caves containing Horseshoe bats within five hundred miles of Wuhan.

The Cover-Up

The market China claimed was the source of the outbreak remained open throughout December despite doctors in Wuhan linking the outbreak there. The market was closed January 1, thirty-one days after the first patient was diagnosed.

The CCP system regards even the most innocuous information to be state secrets that must be protected at all costs. That was the case with information about the coronavirus that was kept secret by China's National Health Commission, the party-controlled group in charge of covering up the virus outbreak.

One of the first patients to be infected was a sixty-five-year-old man who made deliveries to the Wuhan market. He first became sick December 15 and was admitted to Wuhan Central Hospital three days later. His case finally set in motion China's first public notification of the disease outbreak.

On December 24 a bronchial sample from the patient was sent to the Guangzhou Weiyuan Gene Technology Co., Ltd., a medical testing firm. The test results were phoned to the hospital four days later. The results showed that the pathogen was a previously unknown coronavirus.

An anonymous employee who received the sample posted a detailed assessment of it on WeChat. The employee was identified by the economic newspaper *Caixin* under the social media handle "Small Dog." The *Caixin* report was removed by CCP censors, but copies survived through a digital archiving website.

Small Dog recognized immediately that the sample he had assessed involved the discovery of the new virus. On December 27, the complete genome was sequenced. "The information obtained at the time was that this

Two video bloggers who reported inside Wuhan helped show the world the stacks of body bags filled with corpses in the early days of the epidemic.

patient had returned to his hometown and did not rule out contact with bats," the report stated. The writer understood the potential severity of the discovery. To prevent infections, the laboratory was completely cleaned and disinfected. Virus samples were destroyed. Personnel involved in the testing were put on health monitoring, and the patient was quarantined. The genome firm sent officials to Wuhan to notify the hospital and the Wuhan Centers for Disease Control on December 29 and 30. The patient did not survive.

Simultaneously, similar test results from other labs began arriving at hospitals in Wuhan.

At this point, the CCP entered full cover-up mode. The objective was not to protect the people who were being sickened but to limit potential damage to the ruling CCP and most importantly its supreme leader, Xi Jinping.

"Everything is under intense, confidential and strict investigation," the post by Small Dog stated. "At this time, the hospital and the disease control people already know that there are many similar patients. Emergency treatment has been started."

At the same time, an explosion of postings about the new SARS coronavirus detonated in Chinese social media.

For a brief period until CCP censors cracked down, social media provided the first public glimmer of the horror that was to come.

Shortly after a test report on the new coronavirus by the Beijing Boao Medical Laboratory appeared on WeChat on December 30, Li Wenliang, an ophthalmology doctor at Wuhan Central Hospital, sent a message to an online group of friends and medical doctors.

"7 cases of SARS were diagnosed in the South China Fruit and Seafood Market and were isolated in the emergency department of our hospital." Two hours later, Liu Wen, a neurologist, sent a WeChat message to a group of colleagues: "Just after the Second Hospital [Wuhan Central Hospital], a case of coronary infectious viral pneumonia was diagnosed in the Houhu district. SARS has been basically confirmed." The post included a warning to medical workers to adopt protective measures to avoid infection.

Around the same time, Xie Linka, a doctor at the Cancer Center of Wuhan Union Medical College Hospital, posted a WeChat message to an online group of doctors. "Many people have unexplained pneumonia (similar to SARS). Today, our hospital admitted many cases of pneumonia from the Huanan Seafood Market. Everyone should pay attention to wearing masks and ventilation."

A day later, the CCP began censoring all media, including social media, for numerous terms the regime feared were being used to criticize the party, including "Wuhan unknown pneumonia," "SARS variation," "Wuhan Seafood Market," and any other keywords that would signal criticism of the CCP and the government's mishandling of the outbreak.

The reaction by the CCP to the doctors' online warnings was swift. On January 1, eight medical doctors in Wuhan who warned about the new virus outbreak, including Li Wenliang, were detained by security police and interrogated. All were charged with "making false statements on the Internet," a crime in China punishable by imprisonment.

Li was forced to a write what the CCP calls a "self criticism," a tool used by Mao Zedong during his reign as all-powerful dictator for eliminating all vestiges of opposition of the CCP. The doctor was forced to say that his warnings were wrong because they had "a negative impact" on society.

Li, 34, would contract the deadly disease and die on February 7, leaving a pregnant wife and child, who also tested positive for the disease.

He became an instant hero in China for standing up to the party on behalf of the health of its people. His persecution and death set off a wave of anger throughout the population of 1.4 billion people that had not been seen since the bloody Tiananmen Square massacre in June 1989, when People's Liberation Army tanks were called in by the CCP to crush a growing democratic revolt. How could a medical doctor who tried to warn of the impending calamity be so mistreated by a callous and uncaring system? Another of the unanswered questions regarding the crimes of the CCP.

On January 3, Li signed his letter of reprimand telling the Wuhan Public Security Bureau that his posts on WeChat were "illegal."

A month later, in the face of growing popular anger, police rescinded the letter of reprimand but accused the doctor's Chinese supporters of using the "Li Wenliang incident" as part of a conspiracy by "hostile forces" to undermine the CCP leadership.

CCP propagandists sought to turn the tables on popular anger by praising Li as a CCP member they claimed backed the regime. "It should be recognized that certain hostile forces, in order to attack the Chinese Communist Party and the Chinese government, gave Dr. Li Wenliang the label of an anti-system 'hero' and 'awakener.' This is entirely against the facts. Li Wenliang is a Communist Party member, not a so-called 'anti-institutional figure' and those forces with ulterior motives who wish to fan the fires, deceive people and stir up emotions in society are doomed to fail."

"Hostile forces" is the blanket term used

The WHO served as an agent for spreading dangerously false information by the CCP.

by CCP propagandists to discredit those who speak out and criticize party leaders and institutions by insinuating that they are acting as tools for foreign governments.

At the same time the doctors were sounding the alarm, the Hubei health commission ordered all genomics companies to stop testing and to destroy samples. At least nine virus samples has been worked on by the end of December at several testing facilities in China – further spreading the virus around the country. Many of the testing facilities were not told of the dangers or contagiousness of the disease.

Caixin reported that one worker at a gene sequencing firm disclosed that he had received a call on January 1 from an official at the Hubei Provincial Health Commission. The official had said that if any sample of the new virus is sent for testing, it must not be retested and must be destroyed. Information about the sample also must be kept secret from the public. Relevant papers and data on the samples were not to be published in any form.

On January 3, China's National Health Commission issued a notice on "Strengthening the Management of Biological Sample Resources and Related Scientific Research Activities in the Prevention and Control of Major Emergent Infectious Diseases." The directive called for using the strictest security measures possible in handling and transporting the new virus. The objective was to prevent infections in humans and, more important for the CCP, to keep secret all information about the virus.

On January 2, the Wuhan Institute of Virology, the sole laboratory in China capable of working on highly infectious diseases like the new coronavirus, completed the gene sequencing. On January 5 the institute had isolated the virus strain.

Extreme secrecy prevented the genome sequence from being made public until pressure from the international community eventually led the CCP to share it in February.

Another serious misstep occurred in early January when the National Health Commission announced it was sharing the virus genome sequence with the WHO.

Earlier on December 31, Chinese officials, in another egregious example of misinformation, notified WHO country officers in Beijing that the pneumonia in Wuhan was both "preventable and controllable."

Nearly two weeks later, here is what the WHO announced in a statement on the disease outbreak:

WHO is reassured of the quality of the ongoing investigations and the response measures implemented in Wuhan, and the commitment to share information regularly. The evidence is highly suggestive that the outbreak is associated with exposures in one seafood market in Wuhan. The market was closed on 1 January 2020. At this stage, there is no infection among healthcare workers, and no clear evidence of human to human transmission. The Chinese authorities continue their work of intensive surveillance and follow up measures, as well as further epidemiological investigations.

It was a complete lie coated in CCP-style propaganda.

At another point in the statement, the agency said, "WHO does not recommend any specific health measures for travelers."

Later, in a tweet that's still resonating worldwide on social media, the WHO announced that "preliminary investigations conducted by the Chinese authorities have found no clear evidence of human-to-human transmission of the novel #coronavirus (2019-nCoV) identified in #Wuhan, #China."

The Lunar New Year, one of China's largest celebrations, was rapidly approaching at the time of the tweet. It was clear that Xi and the CCP leadership had no intention of limiting travel by tens of millions of Chinese for the coming appropriately named Year of the Rat.

Had authorities in China acted sooner to limit the spread of the virus, as many as 95 percent of the coronavirus cases may have been avoided, according to one British study.

As noted, Wuhan authorities closed the

market on January 1 and began disinfecting the entire area, in the process destroying vital evidence and failing to take blood samples from market workers. The action prevented international investigators from learning which animals at the market may have been carrying the virus. Or did they take those steps because they already knew the source of the virus? Another of the unanswered questions.

Early on in the outbreak, the U.S. Centers for Disease Control and Prevention made repeated requests of both the Chinese government and the WHO to allow American virus experts to go to China. They were stonewalled.

China claimed it notified the United States about the virus, but a senior State Department official said the notification was vague. "No one really picked up on that, and the CDC began asking for access to Wuhan in early January, and it was denied," the official said. "The World Health Organization then asked to bring a team in, and that was denied for about two weeks. And then, when they were finally allowed, they were cooling their heels in Beijing for another two weeks or more."

At the same time, the director of the WHO, Tedros Adhanom Ghebreyesus, an Ethiopian communist who was Beijing's choice to head the organization, offered effusive praise for China's handling of the crisis.

"All the time WHO's Tedros was praising the Chinese for their response, [China's] response was to hide, cover up, and to prevent access to the site where people could have had a better understanding of what was going on," the State Department official said.

On December 31, Taiwan's government, a rival to Beijing, also alerted the WHO based on reports from its sources in China that medical workers were getting sick – a clear sign that the infections were hitting other people not associated with the market and indicating person-to-person transmission.

The information was not published by the WHO's data-sharing platform used by health authorities from 196 countries. Taiwan also alerted Chinese officials, but the warning fell on deaf ears in Beijing.

The WHO, coopted by China through several years of covert influence operations, was first notified by Chinese authorities on December 31 that several cases of pneumonia of unknown origin had broken out.

By January 7, Xi Jinping had taken over the handling of the emerging coronavirus crisis and made perhaps his most serious mistake since taking power in 2012: he made no effort to curtail upcoming holiday travel. By then, the rapidly spreading virus had reached epidemic proportions by asymptomatic carriers. Scores or even hundreds of infected Chinese had become virus time bombs by the beginning of the New Year holiday. They were interspersed among the 4 million to 5 million residents of Wuhan who had left the city and had traveled all over China and the world. That travel would be the beginning of the nightmare pandemic now afflicting nearly every nation on earth.

The doctors were not the only ones who raised a warning early. Chinese writer Wang Fang, known by her pen name Fang Fang, became a voice of opposition against CCP authorities in Wuhan.

She was among the first to expose the Wuhan government's false early claim that the virus could not be transmitted between people and that the disease was preventable and controllable.

"This isn't entirely an issue of moral character, but rather they are a part of a certain machine," she wrote. "The rapid operation of this machine causes their eyes to stare only at their superiors and become unable to see the masses of common people."

By early March, Fang was targeting CCP authorities for their crimes. In a social media post, she wrote, "The government is the people's government; it exists to serve the people. Please take back your arrogance and humbly show gratitude to your masters – the millions of Wuhan people."

The post on March 7 was one of the numerous entries in Fang's book *Diary from a Sealed City* that recounted the mass quarantine that was not imposed on Wuhan until January 23, fifty-two days after the first case was discovered. Fang's posts were quickly censored by authorities but were still able to reach tens of millions of Chinese.

It was clear that Xi and the CCP leadership had no intention of limiting travel by tens of millions of Chinese for the coming appropriately named Year of the Rat.

She was allowed to post her musings on the crisis, but others were not so lucky. Xu Zhangrun, a well-known professor at Tsinghua University, documented the carnage in Wuhan during the quarantine and was silenced by authorities after writing an essay critical of Xi's handling of the virus outbreak.

Two video bloggers who reported inside Wuhan helped show the world the stacks of body bags filled with corpses in the early days of the epidemic.

Both men, Fang Bin and Chen Qiushi, disappeared within days of their postings and are believed to have been imprisoned by CCP security forces.

Their videos went viral and highlighted the growing demand among the Chinese population for free and uncensored speech and press. Under Xi Jinping's dictatorial rule, the limited freedom of expression that existed in the mid 2010s, mainly on vibrant social media outlets in China, had been largely extinguished.

Internal Chinese government documents obtained by the Associated Press exposed the cover-up of the outbreak. The documents revealed that the leader of the National Health Commission, Ma Xiaowei, was aware that China and the world were facing a devastating pandemic on January 14. The documents reveal that senior CCP leaders were also aware of the dangers, including human-to-human transmission, and discussed the threat during a secret conference. Yet the CCP deliberately delayed alerting the world until January 20 – six days that cost lives.

"With the coming of the Spring Festival [Lunar New Year], many people will be traveling, and the risk of transmission and spread is high," the memo continued. "All localities must prepare for and respond to a pandemic."

Instead of locking down the city of Wuhan, thousands of people attended banquets that helped spread the virus, and millions left the city and traveled throughout the world, many carrying the virus.

The documents, provided by a doctor in China, contradict claims by Chinese government spokesmen that China provided information on the disease in an open, transparent and timely manner.

On February 3, Xi Jinping, in a speech to the Politburo Standing Committee, directed CCP organs to "take the initiative to influence international opinion" in shaping the global narrative of the Wuhan coronavirus. Studies concluded that had the public been warned a week earlier to keep distances, wear masks, and restrict travel, the number of infections could have been reduced by two-thirds. And early warning of the outbreak would have saves thousands, perhaps tens of thousands, of lives.

THE DISINFORMATION

By the middle of March, China's cover story about the virus originating in the seafood market was beginning to fray as more information came out about its research into bat coronaviruses, including experiments with viruses capable of infecting humans.

Very early on, a senior American official disclosed to me that shortly after China began its lockdown of Wuhan on January 23, rumors had begun circulating on the Internet that the new virus had been created by the American government and deliberately unleashed in China.

I reported on January 26 in the *Washington Times* that "One ominous sign ... is that false rumors circulating on the Chinese internet claim the virus is part of a U.S. conspiracy to spread germ weapons. That could indicate China is preparing propaganda outlets to counter any charges that the new coronavirus escaped from one of Wuhan's civilian or defense research laboratories."

On March 12 that scenario played out. An official spokesman for the Chinese Ministry of Foreign Affairs, Zhao Lijian, deputy director general of the Foreign Ministry information department, took to Twitter – a social media platform banned in China but open to Chinese propagandists – to spread the anti-U.S. disinformation. Zhao questioned when the first American patient to contract the disease was detected and how many people were infected. "What are the names of the hospitals? It might be U.S. army who brought the epidemic to Wuhan," he wrote, without offering any evidence.

Zhao then urged his followers to read a report produced by a Canadian group called the Centre for Research on Globalization known to publish Russian government disinformation. The spokesman pointed to an article headlined "Further evidence that the virus originated in the U.S."

The spokesman's comments followed the remarks of one of China's most senior virology experts, Zhong Nanshan, who stated during a press conference on February 27 that the new coronavirus may not have originated in China. Instead Zhong suggested that the virus had come from outside the country. He headed the CCP's team of experts investigating the virus. "The infection was first spotted in China," he said. "But the virus may not have originated in China."

The comments by both officials were part of a carefully scripted disinformation campaign designed to deflect growing international outrage at China for its mishandling of the epidemic.

President Trump shot back at the false claim that the U.S. Army had spread the deadly pathogen and began referring publicly to the "Chinese virus," something that so angered Beijing that it prompted a phone call from Xi in late March that produced a temporary truce in the war of words.

White House National Security Adviser Robert O'Brien was the most vocal in denouncing China's handling of the disease outbreak. "This outbreak in Wuhan was covered up," he said in a speech, a cover-up that delayed the global response by two months and led to thousands of deaths.

Beijing also covered up the numbers of people who had died, claiming less than 4,000 had succumbed. But intelligence estimates put the number much higher, with as many as 42,000 dead. And as noted earlier, AEI estimated the number of infections at 2.9 million with 136,000 deaths – at a minimum. Intelligence agencies monitored the exhaust from crematoria in Wuhan and noted that funeral homes were importing 3,500 urns a day, suggesting a horrific death toll.

CONCLUSION

The devastating coronavirus outbreak in China that has made the world sick may have one slightly positive result: it likely will mark the beginning of the end for rule by the Chinese Communist Party. As China expert Minxin Pei put it, the crisis exposed the fragility of Xi Jinping's dictatorial rule. "One likely reason that Beijing failed to take aggressive action to contain the outbreak early on was that few crucial decisions can be made without Xi's direct approval, and he faces heavy demands on his limited time and attention," he wrote in *Foreign Affairs*.

Two of the supreme leader's decisions made after the quarantine of Wuhan – sending an underling to Wuhan instead of visiting himself, dropping out of sight for nearly two weeks – exposed him as a weak and vacillating leader who was late in firing Wuhan's mayor and the provincial leader and slow to prevent the disclosure of the virus in the media.

"The brief window during which Chinese social media and even the official press erupted in outrage revealed just how tenuous the CCP's control over information has become and highlighted the latent power of Chinese civil society," Pei added.

Events revealed the CCP as brittle, not strong, and it bolsters the case for continued pressure and economic decoupling from the People's Republic of China.

"The depth and brazenness of the Chinese Communist Party's lethal mendacity, along with its corruption of WHO, has shocked the international community as if it is something new," said Bernard Moreland, a China expert who once worked at the U.S. Embassy in Beijing.

"Trusting false Chinese data in the early days of this crisis has been lethal for countries foolish enough to do so, including the United States.

*Intelligence agencies monitored
the exhaust from crematoria
in Wuhan and noted that
funeral homes were importing
3,500 urns a day, suggesting
a horrific death toll.*

"There is a sudden moment of clarity about what the CCP really is," Moreland noted. "However it's always been what it is today, an amoral, fundamentally dishonest, relentlessly expansionist and violent bureaucracy. It's primary mission is to extend its own power without limits. Nuisances of governance such as public health, pollution and law enforcement are troublesome distractions to be minimized."

Congress is moving swiftly to hold the CCP accountable with legislation that will seek to punish Beijing for its crimes and force payments for the economic damage, measured in the trillions of dollars.

"This is one of the worst cover-ups in human history, and now the world is facing a global pandemic," said Representative Michael T. McCaul, Texas Republican and ranking member of the House Foreign Affairs Committee.

He and others in Congress have called for investigations into the outbreak. Action with the cooperation of the Trump administration is expected later in 2020 when it is hoped that the epidemic in the United States is under control.

Secretary of State Mike Pompeo promised that China will be held accountable in the future. "There's still lots of work to be done to find out precisely what happened here, precisely how this came to be," he said. "We know this much: We know this is a global pandemic that originated in Wuhan, China. We know that there were wet markets there." China, he said, was too late and too slow in providing information about human-to-human spread of the disease, "and that caused the entire world to be on its back foot at a time when it needed to be leaning forward and moving out aggressively."

Wei Jingsheng, one of China's most prominent political dissidents, bluntly pointed to the Communist Party for its role in the death and disruption caused by the pandemic. The CCP concealed the truth and destroyed evidence to hide the epidemic while promoting the false narrative that the virus could not be transmitted between people. "What was the CCP doing?" Wei said. "This is murder. The use of disease to kill people is an old tradition of the CCP. Initially, it was only aimed at political enemies, but Xi Jinping expanded it against ordinary people across the country."

The virus may not have been engineered by China's bat virologists. But the probability that the virus escaped from a lab in Wuhan is high, and for that the CCP is directly responsible.

The epidemic has altered the political landscape in the United States as the nation is engaged in the 2020 presidential election.

Former Pentagon official Joseph Bosco said the virus has, "serendipitously or otherwise," boosted the fortunes of Xi Jinping and the CCP by ravaging the United States and hitting the American economy hard. Within a few weeks of the U.S. outbreak, 16 million people were out of work, and the stock market plummeted as the country was locked down to limit the spread. "Xi might well have asked his colleagues: Who will rid me of this troublesome president?" Bosco wrote in a column in *The Hill*.

Ben Lowsen, a China expert and adviser to the U.S. military, went further. In an article headlined "Did Xi Jinping Deliberately Sicken the World?", Lowsen argues that the nature of the communist regime is such that it is possible Xi decided to unleash the virus on the world in the hope of weakening the CCP's number-one enemy, the United States.

"We should not assume it was beyond [Xi's] imagining to withhold a degree of support from the international community to ensure that China would not suffer alone," Lowsen wrote in the online magazine *The Diplomat.*

The pandemic caused by China erupted as the United States is moving toward a presidential election. As Vice President Mike Pence has said, China opposes Trump's hardline stance on Chinese trade and other issues and wants a new American president. The comments made in October in a speech included claims that Beijing is covertly working to undermine the Trump administration in hopes of seeing him replaced after the November election. Expect China to exploit the coronavirus epidemic to further the goal of electing a new U.S. president more accommodating to Beijing in 2021.

What Should Be Done

As shown, China's assertion that the virus outbreak was started by poor Chinese peasants mishandling wild animals at a wet market has become increasingly dubious. Strong evidence suggests that the virus set off the pandemic due to poor safety at one of the Wuhan laboratories engaged in studying deadly bat coronaviruses. Proof will no doubt be difficult to obtain from the embattled CCP, which will under all circumstances hide evidence and lie to protect its grip on power.

Nevertheless, the United States, together with the world community, must take action to avoid more deadly epidemics.

As with the Soviet Union's Chernobyl nuclear disaster, the Chinese lied to cover up a major natural disaster – only now the damage is not simply the irradiation of an area in and around a city in Ukraine. The Chinese have inflicted grave damage on the world economy and put half the world's population out of work, at least temporarily.

In response, American policy makers and legislators should debate adopting the following actions and policies:

➤ Friendly U.S. trade and other relations with China must be put on hold and further ties preconditioned on Beijing allowing a major American-led investigation into the origin of the coronavirus. This probe must be carried out without intervention by the WHO or the United Nations. China cannot avoid being held accountable the way Saudi Arabia's government was allowed to avoid scrutiny for its responsibility for the September 11 terrorist attacks.

➤ Congress must act quickly to abolish the sovereign immunity within the U.S. court system for the People's Republic of China and all its tentacles in the United States. Americans must be allowed to obtain the truth and remuneration from China through both civil and criminal legal means.

➤ U.S. policies must be implemented that severely penalize American supply chains and goods that are completely or partially dependent on China. The epidemic revealed that the United States, according to the Food and Drug Administration, is running short of drugs needed to treat coronavirus patients. It turns out that large portions of the U.S. pharmaceutical industry had been moved offshore to China over the past several decades. To bring home the vulnerability this has caused, the CCP threatened at one point to impose exports controls on its pharmaceuticals. The not-so-subtle message from Beijing was that China was ready to plunge the United States into what Chinese state media called "the mighty sea of coronavirus."

> All training in the United States for Chinese managerial, technical, and scientific personnel must be halted immediately. High security laboratories in Wuhan studying deadly pathogens are staffed by Western-trained and Western-educated personnel. The pandemic demonstrated that China's ruling CCP system cannot be trusted to be the "responsible stake-

holder" several U.S. presidential administrations tried to produce with conciliatory policies that included the influx of hundreds of thousands of Chinese nationals. American universities and research institutes have become too dependent on CCP cash. They must find alternatives and must be barred from working with PRC students and researchers.

> To counter the CCP's covert infiltration and takeover of international organizations like the WHO, the United States must expel the People's Republic of China from international organizations. Alternatively, the United States should withdraw from international organizations under Beijing's control. CCP control over the WHO resulted in Chinese leaders' complicity in mass death. It must never be repeated. Expelling China from the World Trade Organization is also needed because the promised reforms its mem-

bership in the organization were supposed to produce in the Chinese system didn't take place. The United States should reform such organizations by working solely with like-minded democracies.

It is now clear that decades of international engagement and cooperation with Communist China was a mistake that seriously undermined fundamental American values of freedom, democracy, openness, honesty, and free markets.

A state that has imprisoned more than 1 million of its citizens in concentration camps in western China and supplied nuclear

---

Scores or even hundreds of infected Chinese had become virus time bombs by the beginning of the New Year holiday.

---

weapons technology and long-range missile equipment to American enemies like North Korea and Iran should no longer be part of the U.S.-led free world order.

The world does not need to prove that the Communist regime in Beijing was responsible for the escape of the coronavirus from a lab or that it allowed the continued operation of potentially deadly wild animal markets. We know enough about the nefarious behavior of the Chinese Communist Party to put these national defense and security measures into place. The time to act is now.

First American edition published in 2020 by Encounter Books,
an activity of Encounter for Culture and Education, Inc.,
a nonprofit, tax exempt corporation.
Encounter Books website address: www.encounterbooks.com

Manufactured in the United States and printed on
acid-free paper. The paper used in this publication meets
the minimum requirements of ANSI / NISO Z39.48–1992
(R 1997) (*Permanence of Paper*).

FIRST AMERICAN EDITION

LIBRARY OF CONGRESS CATALOGING-IN-PUBLICATION DATA
IS AVAILABLE